CW00458732

PRESCRIPTION DRUGS

PRESCRIPTION DRUGS

Dr D G Delvin

MB BS LRCP MRCS DOBST
RCOG DCH FPA CERT
MRCGP DIP VEN

The ROYAL
SOCIETY of
MEDICINE

SUNBURST BOOKS

Editorial Advisor

DR KATHARINE A ORTON
MB BS MRCGP
DCH DRCOG

Author's Acknowledgement
Many thanks to Jo Grimes, MR Pharm S,
for her help with this book

This edition first published in 1995 by
Sunburst Books, Deacon House,
65 Old Church Street, London SW3 5BS.

Copyright
Text © David Delvin 1995
Layout and design © Sunburst Books 1995

ISBN 1 85778 164 3

Printed and bound in China

CONTENTS

INTRODUCTION

This quick-reference guide to prescription drugs includes all the pills, tablets and medicines which are most likely to be prescribed by your doctor when you are ill.

This booklet is not intended to replace your doctor's advice but to augment it. When she or he prescribes medication for you:

Ask her or him for information about the drug and its possible side-effects.

If you have any further queries, put them to your pharmacist when you collect the prescription from her or him. In many countries, pharmacists now have a wealth of information available about medications and their possible interactions with other drugs – on a computer database.

At all costs, read the label carefully. If there is a leaflet from the manufacturer, read that too, despite the fact that some contain technical jargon and may be written in very fine print.

Finally, look up your medication in this book. If there is anything you still don't understand, check again with your own physician to ensure that you are taking the medicine safely and effectively.

WARNINGS

Please read these warnings carefully.

Side Effects All drugs can have side-effects. In fact, many drugs have hundreds of them. This book indicates some of the most common side-effects of each medication. If you have *any* untoward side effect while on a drug, please do check with your doctor.

Drug Interactions Many drugs can 'interact' with other drugs to produce unwanted results. So make sure that the doctor who prescribes for you knows what other drugs you are taking.

Pregnancy If you are pregnant, it's usually best not to take any medication at all, unless your doctor feels it is absolutely necessary. Therefore, make sure that any physician whom you consult is aware of the fact that you are pregnant.

Alcohol While on any medication, it is usually best to avoid alcohol unless your doctor has said it is safe to take a drink. Some drugs, particularly sedatives, are very dangerous with alcohol.

Driving Many drugs, such as tranquillisers, make people slightly sleepy and interfere with their co-ordination and their speed of reaction. If there is the least reason to suspect that you could be affected, do not drive.

We hope that this book will be useful to you and your family, and will help you get the very best out of your doctor's treatment.

Dr David Delvin

CLASSES OF DRUGS

Entries in this quick-reference book will sometimes refer you to one of the classes of drugs listed below:

ACE-INHIBITORS

This group of drugs is useful in high blood pressure (hypertension), and in heart failure. 'Heart failure' does not mean that the heart has stopped beating. It means that it's not working as well as it should, so that, for instance, fluid is accumulating in the body's tissues.

ACE-inhibitors work by preventing the formation of a natural body chemical called 'angiotensin II'. This closes down the small tubes through which blood flows, keeping the blood pressure up, and making it harder for the heart to work.

The chief side effects of the various ACE-inhibitors are mentioned under their individual entries. However, it is worth noting that in general they can cause faintness due to low blood pressure, dry cough, throat discomfort, voice changes, tiredness and loss of taste.

ANTACIDS

These are drugs which are meant to neutralise the acid produced in your stomach, since excess acid can cause indigestion pain or heartburn and is also associated with ulcers. They are useful in a common condition called 'reflux oesophagitis', in which there is inflammation of the lower end of the gullet.

Antacids are probably best given when pain occurs or when it is expected, unless your doctor says otherwise. Very often, she or he will suggest that you take them between meals and/or just before going to bed, because acid output is usually high during the night.

Do not take antacids with other medication, because they may interfere with the absorption of other drugs.

ANTIBIOTICS

Antibiotics are drugs which are useful against bacteria. They have no effect on viruses, such as those which cause colds.

It is important not to use them unnecessarily, so don't put pressure on your doctor to prescribe one if she or he does not think it appropriate.

There are various different groups of antibiotics:

Penicillins The penicillins were the first of the antibiotics and are still very useful, although many bacteria have developed resistance to them. They work by attacking the building-blocks of the germs' cell walls.

Unfortunately, many people are sensitive to these drugs and develop a severe and irritating rash when they are prescribed. If you are penicillin-sensitive, take care to mention the fact to every doctor you consult during your life. Carrying the information in your purse or wallet is well worthwhile, especially as a few penicillin-sensitive people are hit by a life-threatening collapse if given one of these drugs.

Cephalosporins These antibiotics are useful against a wide range of bacteria, and work in much the same way as the penicillins.

Unfortunately, cephalosporins too can produce sensitivity reactions, and about one in ten of people who are sensitive to penicillins are also sensitive to cephalosporins.

Tetracyclines These antibiotics attack a wide range of germs, but unfortunately many bacteria are resistant to them these days. They also stain growing teeth very badly, and therefore must not be given to children or pregnant women. They can cause sickness and diarrhoea, and may interfere with your absorption of other drugs, including the contraceptive pill.

Do not take milk or antacids with tetracyclines; you will not absorb the antibiotic properly. If you have kidney disease, you should not be on most tetracyclines.

ANTI-DEPRESSANTS

These are drugs which are designed to lift the mood in depressive illness. Many people confuse them with tranquillisers, such as Valium and Librium, but in fact they are not related in any way at all.

Anti-depressants work by altering the levels of concentration of various natural brain chemicals, since it is thought that an imbalance of these chemicals lies behind most cases of depression.

They are not at all addictive, as some patients fear, but they are powerful agents and it is very important that you stick to the dose that your physician has prescribed. It is also vital that you keep these potentially lethal drugs out of the hands of any children in your home.

ANTI-HISTAMINES

These are drugs which work against allergies. They are effective because they counteract the effects of histamine, a rather troublesome body chemical which is released from cells in cases of allergic reaction.

Older anti-histamines have the disadvantage of making people sleepy, which is not only a nuisance at exam times, but also poses a real threat to safety if a person drives or operates machinery. Some newer anti-histamines are relatively free of this risk.

BETA-BLOCKERS

This group of drugs was invented in the 1960s. They are useful in high blood pressure, angina (heart pain caused by narrowing of the coronary arteries), after a heart attack, and in certain other conditions, including anxiety. They work in a complex way which involves blocking little 'receptors' into which the molecules of certain body chemicals would normally fit.

Some beta-blockers are 'heart selective', which means that they are less likely to produce effects in organs other than the heart. Such effects are likely to be undesirable.

All beta-blockers can narrow the air tubes and cause wheezing, so there is danger in taking them if you have asthma, emphysema or chronic bronchitis.

CALCIUM ANTAGONISTS

These drugs, often called 'calcium-channel blockers' are useful in angina, high blood pressure, and many cases of irregular heartbeat.

They work by a very complicated action, involving interference with the way that calcium travels through the walls of cells in your heart and in the muscle contained in blood vessels.

Calcium antagonists vary a great deal in their side-effects: see individual entries. They should not be stopped suddenly, as this might cause angina attacks.

DIURETICS

Often known as 'water pills', these are drugs that make you pass more urine. This is a useful property, especially where a person's body is 'water-logged', as, for instance, in heart failure. However, diuretics are no use as slimming aids. They get rid of water, not fat.

Diuretics work by means of various complex effects on the kidney, which is the organ that filters the blood and expels waste products in the form of urine.

Unfortunately, all diuretics can cause major imbalances in the body's mineral balance – very frequently, the balance of potassium. So these drugs are never prescribed by doctors without careful thought.

Very often, it's necessary to have regular blood tests, to make sure that the levels of your blood minerals, particularly potassium, are satisfactory.

Potassium chloride is prescribed at the same time as many diuretics in order to keep the blood level of potassium up to normal (see **potassium chloride**).

LAXATIVES

Laxatives (aperients) are much less often prescribed by doctors than they used to be, which is why there are very few of them in this book. Physicians now believe that daily bowel movements are not essential for good health. Furthermore, today's medical opinion is that taking plenty of natural fibre in the diet is much preferable to taking drugs, especially as many laxatives have the capacity to numb the bowel through long-term use so that it ceases to function properly.

In general, you should take a laxative only if your physician advises it. Sudden constipation occurring in the middle-aged and elderly should be reported to a doctor urgently, rather than treated with laxatives.

NSAIDs

This increasingly commonly-used abbreviation stands for 'Non-Steroidal Anti-Inflammatory Drugs'. This term covers the very large number of compounds which are used against arthritis, rheumatic disorders and pain in the bones, joints and muscle. They are also becoming widely and successfully used against period pain. They combat inflammation as well as pain.

You can really regard this group of drugs as 'aspirin and its modern successors'. They work by preventing the formation of natural 'pain and inflammation agents', called prostaglandins.

It is an unfortunate fact that nearly all NSAIDs can have serious adverse effects, particularly on the stomach and intestines. They cause irritation and may induce abdominal discomfort,

nausea, diarrhoea and occasionally ulcers
or internal bleeding.

Do not take aspirin or other NSAIDs if you have
an active ulcer. If you have had an ulcer in the
past, you should only take NSAIDs if your
physician feels that the benefit substantially
outweighs the risk.
Do not take any NSAIDs if you have a history of
hypersensitivity to aspirin, or any other member
of this group. In particular, do not take them if
you have ever had an attack of asthma provoked
by aspirin or any NSAID.

NSAIDs must be used with extreme caution
in the elderly and in people with kidney, heart or
liver problems. Be guided by your own doctor as
to whether they are suitable for you.

OPIATES

Opiates are powerful painkillers. They are all
related to opium and heroin.

They are very effective in easing pain, but their
big drawback is that the stronger ones, such as
morphine, will make almost anyone addicted
within quite a short time. Therefore, repeated
administration is best avoided.

Opiates work by mimicking the action of certain
natural painkillers in the brain. Unfortunately, with
repeated administration it is often the case that
larger doses are required to produce the same
painkilling effect.

Side-effects of opiates include drowsiness,
sickness and constipation. Larger doses may
cause suppression of adequate breathing, which
may be serious, particularly in older people.

STEROIDS

Steroids are drugs related to cortisone, the natural anti-inflammatory body chemical.

There are various different types of steroid, but the ones which are most commonly prescribed have the effect of 'damping down' inflammation. This makes them useful in such conditions as:

* Asthma

* Allergies

* Various types of arthritis (but not 'ordinary' arthritis, osteoarthritis)

* Eczema (dermatitis) and other inflammatory skin conditions

* Inflammatory bowel disorders, such as ulcerative colitis.

Regrettably, although steroids can have dramatic healing actions, the fact is that when taken by mouth or injected they can have very serious – sometimes even life-threatening – side-effects. They can, for example, cause:

* Ulcers   * High blood pressure

* Growth stunting   * Thinning of the bones

* Diabetes   * Mental disturbances

* Spread of infection in the body.

Therefore, doctors prescribe oral and injectable steroids only sparingly. Steroids applied to the skin can also have unfortunate effects such as permanent red marks, or thinning of skin layers, so these must be used strictly in accordance with your doctor's instructions.

Oral steroids should never be stopped abruptly; they must be 'tailed off' gradually. Again, this should be as prescribed by your physician. Inhaled steroids are used very widely for asthma. Many people fear that they will have the serious side-effects of oral steroids, but this isn't the case. When inhaled, the anti-asthma steroids are remarkably free from dangerous effects.

TRANQUILLISERS

These are drugs which calm a person down and ease anxiety. They do this by a sedative action on the brain.

It is a fact of life that vast numbers of people now take tranquillisers, although many physicians believe that they are often taken unnecessarily.

Regrettably, nearly all tranquillisers eventually prove to be habit-forming. Once you are 'hooked', it is very difficult to get off a tranquilliser, and you may have quite unpleasant symptoms if you try to stop. Therefore, medical authorities now advise that tranquillisers should only be taken for short periods, and when absolutely necessary.

Many of them will impair co–ordination, and hence driving skills. Unless you are sure that your reaction speeds and co-ordination are normal, do not drive or operate machinery or computers.

A-Z

OF

PRESCRIPTION
DRUGS

Acebutolol

One of the 'beta-blocker' group of drugs *(see **Classes of Drugs***). Used in treating high blood pressure (hypertension), angina, and irregular heart rhythm (for method of action and possible side-effects *see **beta-blockers** under **Classes of Drugs**).*

Acebutolol is one of the 'cardio-selective' beta-blockers, meaning that its action is concentrated upon the heart, so that adverse effects elsewhere in the body are less likely. Trade names include Sectral

Acepril Trade name for captopril

Acetaminophen *see **paracetamol***

Achromycin Trade name for tetracycline

Acyclovir

One of the few effective anti-virus drugs available. Works by interfering with the synthesis of DNA. Used in the treatment of herpes of the mouth, of the eye or the genitals, and also against shingles, which are all viral infections. Works only if treatment is started as early as possible. It is unlikely to be of use after the attack has started.

Possible side-effects include:
Cream: redness and flaking of the skin
By mouth: tummy upsets, rashes, headache, tiredness, blood changes
Trade names include Zovirax

Adalat Trade name for nifedipine

Adizem Trade name for diltiazem

Aerobec Trade name for beclomethasone

Aerolin Trade name for salbutamol

Allegron Trade name for nortriptyline

Allopurinol
Allopurinol is a drug used against gout, purely on a long-term basis. It must not be used to treat an acute attack, since it could make this worse.

It works by affecting an enzyme within the body, so as to reduce production of uric acid, raised levels of which cause gout.

Possible side-effects include nausea and skin reactions, and also attacks of gout in the early days of treatment.
Trade names include Zyloric, Lopurin, Zurinol, Zyloprim, Hamarin

Aludrox Trade name for aluminium hydroxide

Aluminium hydroxide
One of the 'antacid' group of drugs *(see **Classes of Drugs**)*. Useful in conditions of excess stomach acid, indigestion and ulcers. Works by the neutralisation of excess acid. Usually best taken between meals and/or at bedtime. Do not take at the same time as other drugs, as they may not be properly absorbed. Avoid if you have glaucoma, or if you have a low level of phosphate in your blood.

Possible side effects include constipation.
Trade names include Aludrox

Alupent Trade name for orciprenaline

Amfipen Trade name for ampicillin

Aminophylline
Widens the air passages, so making breathing easier. It is useful in asthma, emphysema, and chronic bronchitis.

Possible side-effects include nausea, irritation of the stomach and wakefuness.
Trade names include Phyllocontin, Pecram, Amoline, Somophyllin

Amitriptyline
One of the 'anti-depressant' group of drugs *(see* **Classes of Drugs***)*. Prescribed in order to try and lift the mood in cases of depression. Like other similar anti-depressants, works mainly by prolonging the active life of two natural chemicals in the brain, noradrenalin and serotonin. The full mechanism of action is not known at present. Unlike some other anti-depressants, has a sedative effect and may promote sleep.

Possible side-effects include dry mouth, blurred vision, constipation, difficulty in passing urine, palpitations, tremor, dizziness, sweating, fatigue.
Trade names include Tryptizol, Lentizol, Amitril, Elavil, Emitrip, Endep

Amoram Trade name for amoxycillin

Amoxil Trade name for amoxycillin

Amoxycillin
An antibiotic of the penicillin group *(see* **antibiotics** *under* **Classes of Drugs***)*. Amoxycillin is a penicillin of the type described as 'broad spectrum' because it hits a wide range of germs.

It is useful in ear and sinus infections, urinary infections, and flare-ups of chronic bronchitis.

Possible side-effects include bowel disturbances and skin reactions due to hypersensitivity.
Trade names include Amoxil, Amoram, Flemoxin, Galenamox, Larotid, Polymox, Trimox, Utimox, Wymox

Ampicillin

One of the penicillin group of antibiotics *(see antibiotics under Classes of Drugs)*.

A broad spectrum penicillin which attacks many different types of germ. Particularly used against infections of the ear, nose, throat and chest, cystitis and gonorrhoea.

It must under no circumstances be given if the person could have glandular fever (infectious mononucleosis, or 'mono'), because it will cause a severe and very irritating skin eruption.

Otherwise, possible side effects include stomach disturbances and – in cases of hypersensitivity to penicillins – a skin rash.
Trade names include Penbritin, Amfipen, Amcil, D-Amp, Omnipen, Polycillin, Principen, Totacillin

Anafranil Trade name for clomipramine

Angettes Trade name for aspirin

Antabuse Trade name for disulfiram

Artane Trade name for benxhexol

Ascorbic acid *see vitamin C*

Aspirin

Although aspirin is available over the counter, doctors frequently write prescriptions for it. It is useful for treating headaches, colds, muscle pains, rheumatism, period pain, and various types of arthritis. In addition to its pain-relieving qualities, it has a powerful anti-inflammatory effect, and helps lower a raised temperature.

However, it should not be given to children because it is believed to increase the risk of a rare but very serious childhood ailment called Reye's syndrome. In all age groups, over-dosage is extremely dangerous.

Possible side-effects of aspirin include stomach ache, internal bleeding, wheezing, and ringing in the ears. It can also help prevent your blood from clotting, although there are certain circumstances where this can be a good thing, for instance, in cases of heart attack.

Astemizole

One of the anti-histamine drugs (see **anti-histamines** under **Classes of Drugs).** Used for hay fever, dust mite allergy, other forms of allergic nose inflammation, and for allergic skin conditions. Astermizole is rather slower than other similar drugs in taking effect. Unlike older anti-histamines, it is claimed not to cause sleepiness; however, use caution if driving or operating machinery.

Possible side-effects include occasional weight gain and, **very importantly,** heart irregularities in certain circumstances. So read the label with even more care than usual, and never exceed the stated dose.

Trade names include Hismanal

Atenolol

A 'beta-blocker' drug, used for the treatment of angina, pulse irregularities and raised blood pressure. For mode of action and possible side-effects, *see **beta-blockers** under **Classes of Drugs***.

Atenolol is specifically designed to target the heart, so it is rather less likely than some other beta-blockers to cause unwanted effects elsewhere. Being one of a group of beta-blockers which are 'water-soluble', it is relatively free of side-effects on the brain, such as sleep disturbances and nightmares.
Trade names include Tenormin, Totamol

Atromid-S Trade name for clofibrate

Augmentin

Trade name for a widely prescribed combination of amoxycillin *(see **amoxycillin**)* and clavulanic acid, a weak antibiotic which 'augments' the effect of the other ingredient. Used in respiratory infections, and also infections of the ear, urinary tract, skin and soft tissues.

Possible side-effects are those of amoxycillin.

Aventyl Trade name for nortriptyline

Avloclor Trade name for chloroquine

Avomine Trade name for promethazine

Azapropazone

A non-steroidal anti-inflammatory agent or NSAID *(see NSAID under **Classes of Drugs**).* Like other NSAIDs, azapropazone has the valuable property of reducing inflammation, therefore often reducing pain. However, its use is now mainly restricted to treating rheumatoid arthritis and ankylosing spondylitis – and also acute gout, where other remedies have failed.

Possible side-effects, which are not shared by most other members of this drug group, include excessive sensitivity of the skin to sunlight. Also possible are internal bleeding, waterlogging of the tissues and blood abnormalities. The drug must not be taken by anyone who has had an ulcer. Trade names include Rheumox

Bactrim Trade name for co-trimoxazole

Baxan Trade name for cefadroxil

Beclazone Trade name for beclomethasone

Becloforte Trade name for beclomethasone

Beclomethasone
Valuable inhaled steroid (see **inhaled steroids** in **Classes of Drugs**).

It is used to treat hay fever and asthma, because it dampens down inflammation. For hay fever, a nasal aerosol or atomiser is employed, in order to deposit the drug in the nose passages. It is of no use in treating an attack, but has to be taken over a long-term period.

For asthma, the drug is administered by inhalation of an aerosol through the mouth, or by inhalation of a dry powder or a nebulised suspension. Again, the drug must be used long-term to gain maximum benefit.

Possible side-effects include hoarseness, attacks of thrush in the mouth and thinning of bones. However beclomethasone seems to be free of the risks of growth-stunting associated with oral steroid drugs.
Trade names include Beclazone, Aerobec, Becloforte, Becodisks, Becotide, Filair, Beconase, Beclovent, Vancenase, Vanceril

Benoral Trade name of benorylate

Benorylate
A non-steroidal anti-inflammatory drug (see **NSAIDs, in Classes of Drugs**). Benorylate is a close relation of both aspirin and paracetamol. It is mainly used to treat osteoarthritis (osteoarthosis), rheumatoid arthritis, and other causes of pain in the muscles or joints. It works by damping down inflammation, and thus reducing pain and swelling.

Possible side-effects are those of aspirin and paracetamol. It should **not** be given to children.
Trade names include Benoral

Benzhexol
Anti-Parkinson's disease drug. Useful in reducing trembling, stiffness and dribbling. Works by altering the balance of 'nerve transmitter' chemicals in the brain.

Possible side-effects include dry mouth, blurred vision, tummy upsets, dizziness, difficulty in passing urine, confusion and nervousness.
Trade names include Artane, Broflex

Betahistine
A drug which is marketed as a treatment for Ménière's disease because it helps to reduce

dizziness and other symptoms associated with this disabling condition.

The mode of action is not yet clearly understood. Possible side-effects are intestinal disturbances, headache, rashes and itching.
Trade names include Serc

Betaloc Trade name for metoprolol

Betamethasone
A powerful steroid drug (see **steroids** under **Classes of Drugs**), which is used to treat severe asthma, rheumatic arthritis, collagen (connective tissue) diseases and some allergic conditions. Works by damping down inflammatory conditions.

Possible side-effects are similar to those of other steroids (see **Classes of Drugs**); since they may be serious, it is vitally important to stick to your doctor's instructions.
Trade names include Betnelan, Betnesol

Betim Trade name for timolol

Biorphen Trade name for orphenadrine

Bismuth chelate
Anti-ulcer preparation. This agent has been increasingly used, together with two antibiotics, to try to eradicate the germ *Helicobacter pylori*, which is thought by one school of doctors to be responsible for many ulcers.

Side-effects include dark tongue, black motions, nausea.
Trade names include De-Nol, De-Noltab

Bisoprolol

A 'beta-blocker' drug *(see **Beta-blockers** under* ***Classes of Drugs)***. Prescribed in the treatment of raised blood pressure and angina. The mode of action and side-effects are similar to those of other beta-blockers and are described under Classes of Drugs. Bisoprolol is heart-selective, which means that it is rather less likely to cause ill-effects in other parts of the body.
Trade names include Emcor, Monocor

Blocadren Trade name for timolol

Bolvidon Trade name for mianserin

Bricanyl Trade name for diltiazem

Broflex Trade name for benzhexol

Brompheniramine

Anti-histamine (s*ee **anti-histamines** under* ***Classes of Drugs)***. Prescribed in the treatment of hay fever, urticaria and other allergies. For mode of action and possible side-effects, please see ***Classes of Drugs***. Note especially that brompheniramine is a sedative, and because of the risk of drowsiness should not be taken if driving or using machinery.
Trade names include Dimotane, Bromphen, Diamine TD, Dimetane, Veltane

Buccastem Trade name for prochlorperazine.

Buprenorphine

One of the 'opiate' drugs (s*ee **opiates** under* ***Classes of Drugs)***. A very powerful pain-killer, with similar possible side-effects to those of other opiates. Note that withdrawal symptoms

may occur when you stop using it.
Trade names include Temgesic

Calpol Trade name for paracetamol

Camcolit Trade name for lithium carbonate

Caprin
An aspirin preparation (see **aspirin**). Used in rheumatic conditions, and in the prevention of heart attacks. For possible side-effects, see **aspirin**.

Captopril
One of the ACE-inhibitor group of drugs (see **ACE-inhibitors** under **Classes of Drugs,** for mode of action and possible side-effects). Used in mild to moderate hypertension (raised blood pressure) and some cases of severe hypertension. Also used in heart failure and following heart attacks.
Trade names include Acepril, Capoten

Carace Trade name for lisinopril

Carbamazepine
Useful multi-purpose drug, prescribed in the treatment of epilepsy, in relieving the severe pain of trigeminal neuralgia ('tic douloureux') and also in helping people with manic depression.

Possible side-effects include intestinal upsets, skin rashes, blood problems and jaundice.
Trade names include Tegretol

Carbimazole
Drug used to treat overactivity of the thyroid gland (thyrotoxicosis; hyperthyroidism). Works by

interfering with the formation of thyroid hormone.
It is a useful alternative to (a) having the thyroid
gland removed by surgery; or (b) having
radiotherapy to the gland.

Possible side-effects include skin rashes,
headaches, feeling sick and joint pains. Most
importantly, carbimazole can sometimes cause
serious blood disorders, the first signs of which
may be sore throats or mouth ulcers. If you get
either of these symptoms, it is vital to contact
your doctor immediately.
Trade names include Neo-Mercazole

Cardene Trade name for nicardipine

Cedocard Trade name for isosorbide dinitrate

Cefaclor, Cefadroxil, Cefixime, Cephalexin, Cephradine
These are all members of the 'cephalosporin'
group of antibiotics (see **antibiotics** under
Classes of Drugs).

Ceporex Trade name for cephalexin

Chendol see **chenodeoxycholic acid**

Chenix see **chenodeoxycholic acid**

Chenodeoxycholic acid
Drug used to treat certain types of gallstone,
avoiding the need for an operation. It works
by dissolving the stones. It is only effective
against small stones, of a variety called
'radiolucent'. Chenodeoxycholic acid does
not work in people whose gall bladders are
not functioning.

Possible side-effects include colicky pain,
diarrhoea and skin itching.
Trade names include Chendol, Chenofalk, Chenix

Chenofalk *see chenodeoxycholic acid*

Chloral
Also known as 'chloral hydrate', this is a
traditional remedy for sleeplessness. As with
most sedatives, drowsiness may continue next
day and affect driving or machine operation.
Possible side-effects include stomach irritation,
wind, and excitement instead of sleepiness.
Trade names include Welldorm, Noctec,
Aquachloral Supprettes

Chloramphenicol
An antibiotic *(see **antibiotics** in Classes of
Drugs)*. Although it is a powerful agent against
certain germs, chloramphenicol is now not much
used in Western countries except as an eye –
and sometimes skin – application. This is
because of the fact that when taken by mouth it
carries a very high risk of causing serious blood
disorders. However, it remains a very useful drug
in the treatment of the tropical/semi-tropical
illness, typhoid fever.
Trade names include Chloromycetin

Chlordiazepoxide
Tranquilliser (*see **tranquillisers** under Classes of
Drugs).* Under the world-wide trade name
'Librium', this was one of the most consumed
drugs of the 1960s and 1970s, and it is still
used on quite a wide scale.

It acts by damping down brain activity, thus
lessening anxiety. This long-lasting sedative
effect, which may persist till next day, slows the

brain's reactions and may well impair driving and the operation of machinery, or make complex tasks difficult to perform.

Most importantly, this drug – like others of the 'benzodiapine' group, such as diazepam – will make most people 'hooked' if taken for any length of time. Trying to stop it may be very difficult and distressing.

Various national bodies now recommend that the drug is not to be taken for more than a period of two to four weeks. It is important to come off this drug gradually, otherwise severe withdrawal symptoms may occur.

Trade names include Librium, Libritabs, Lipoxide, A-poxide, Mitran, Murcil, Reposans-10

Chloromycetin *see chloramphenicol*

Chloroquine

Principally used as an antimalarial drug, but also used to treat rheumatoid arthritis and the tropical infection amoebic dysentery.

Chloroquine is used both for the treatment and prevention of malaria. It works by interfering with the metabolism of the malaria parasite.

There is now a great deal of malarial resistance to chloroquine in many parts of the world. So it is usually best not take it to protect yourself against malaria unless you have been given expert advice that it is the right drug for the area of the globe where you're going.

In many tropical regions, it needs to be combined with other drugs to give effective protection. Possible side-effects include stomach upsets,

headache, skin rashes, eye problems and
sometimes blood disorders.
Trade names include Avloclor, Nivaquine

Chlorpheniramine
Anti-histamine (*see **anti-histamines** under
Classes of Drugs). Used for allergic conditions.
This is one of the older, sedative anti-histamines,
so it does make people drowsy and slows
reactions, so do not use it if you are driving,
operating machinery, or doing anything which will
require swift reactions. Newer, non-sedative
anti-histamines are now available.
Trade names include Piriton, Chlor-Pro,
Chlorspan, Teldrin

Chlorpromazine
A very powerful tranquilliser, mainly used in
schizophrenia and other severe psychological
disturbances. Works by sedating the brain.

Possible side-effects include drowsiness, apathy,
paleness, depression and sometimes odd
movements of the tongue and face which may
give the misleading impression that more of the
drug is needed. Withdrawal can be very difficult.

Warning: because of the high risk of 'contact
sensitisation', health workers and patients'
relatives should try to avoid direct contact with
this drug. In particular, don't crush tablets up
with your fingers.
Trade names include Largactil, Thorazine,
Promapar, Sonazine, Thor-Prom

Chlorpropamide
Drug used in treating the type of diabetes which
does not require insulin injections.

Chlorpropamide tablets work by stimulating the person's pancreas to produce natural insulin, and by increasing the effect of insulin on the body. The tablets must be used in combination with a carefully prescribed diet.

Possible side-effects include flushing of the face after alcohol consumption, skin rashes and excessively low blood sugar.
Trade names include Diabinese

Cholestyramine
Cholesterol-lowering agent, also sometimes used as a treatment for unusual types of diarrhoea. Works by reducing the levels of 'bile acids' in the body. Mainly used in middle-aged males who have very high cholesterol levels which are not responding to a strict diet.

Side-effects may include constipation, the aggravation of piles, and a tendency to bleed.
Trade names include Questran, Questran Light

Cimetidine
Effective drug against ulcers, and certain other conditions involving excess acid production, such as reflux oesophagitis. Became famous in the 1980s under the trade name Tagamet. Works by reducing your stomach's gastric acid output.

Side-effects may include mild diarrhoea, dizziness, rashes, tiredness and headache. Both men and women may get slightly swollen breasts. Impotence is a rare complication.
Trade names include Tagamet, Dispamet, Galenamet, Zita

Cinnarizine
Anti-nausea agent. Works by 'damping down'

brain centres. Can be taken before travel, but do not drive or operate machinery.

Possible side-effects include drowsiness, skin reactions, and occasionally abnormal movements of the muscles.
Trade names include Stugeron

Ciprofloxacin
Antibiotic *(see **antibiotics** under **Classes of Drugs**)*. A relatively new antibiotic which is used on a wide scale against urinary, respiratory, ear, skin and soft tissue infections. Works by attacking life systems of bacteria.

Possible side-effects include nausea, abdominal pain, diarrhoea, dizziness, headache, rashes.
Trade names include Ciproxin

Ciproxin *see **ciprofloxacin***

Clarithromycin
An antibiotic (see **antibiotics** under **Classes of Drugs**). Fairly recently introduced, this drug is used against respiratory and skin infections and also earache.

Possible side-effects include nausea, diarrhoea, tummy ache and rashes.
Trade names include Klaricid

Clofibrate
Drug which lowers cholesterol and other blood fats in patients whose high blood fat levels have not responded to strict dietary treatment. It is still not understood exactly how it does this.

Possible side-effects include gallstones and muscle inflammation. Therefore, in some

countries it is only given to people who have had their gall-bladders removed. Some studies have shown an increased death rate with long-term use, so ask your physician to keep you informed of any new developments.
Trade names include Atromid-S

Clomiphene
Fertility drug used for ovulation problems. Induces the hypothalamus, a structure at the base of the brain, to increase stimulation of the ovary, and thus egg production.

If the drug works, there is an increased chance of multiple birth. Side-effects may include: eye problems, hot flushes, tummy ache, enlargement of the ovaries.
Trade names include Clomid, Serophene

Clomipramine
Anti-depressant *(see **anti-depressants** under **Classes of Drugs**)*. A drug which has been used for many years to try to lift the mood in depression. Works by increasing the amount of the natural chemicals noradrenaline and serotonin in the brain.

Possible side-effects include dry mouth, blurred vision, constipation and difficulty in urinating.
Trade names include Anafranil

Clonazepam
Drug used against epilepsy. Related to the common tranquillisers, clonazepam works by damping down excessive electrical activity in the brain, thus helping to prevent fits.

Possible side-effects include drowsiness, confusion and giddiness. People do readily

become 'hooked' on this group of drugs They must not be stopped suddenly, since fits and/or withdrawal symptoms may result.
Trade names include Rivotril, Clonopin

Codeine
Pain reliever; also useful in easing diarrhoea, and sometimes as a cough suppressant. Although people think of codeine as a mild over-the-counter drug, it is actually a relative of morphine. In the form prescribed by doctors, it is effective in fighting mild to moderate pain.

Side-effects may include light-headedness, sleepiness, constipation.

Convulex Trade name for valproic acid

Coracten Trade name for nifedipine

Cordilox Trade name for verapamil

Co-trimoxazole
Anti-infection drug, much used in the 1980s world-wide under the trade names Bactrim, Septrin and Septra, for cystitis and other urinary tract infections, chronic bronchitis, and prostate gland inflammation.

Co-trimoxazole consists of a mixture of two drugs: trimethoprim *(see **trimethoprim**)* and a sulphonamide drug called 'sulphamethoxazole', which help each other to fight bacteria.

Side-effects may include sore or ulcerated mouth and tongue, nausea, rashes (some severe) and blood disorders.

Cupanol Trade name for paracetamol

Cyclopenthiazide

Drug that makes you pass more urine *(see diuretics under Classes of Drugs)*. Used in heart failure, oedema (edema; dropsy), and in high blood pressure. Works by encouraging the kidneys to allow more urine through.

Possible side-effects include disturbance in body minerals, tummy upsets, rashes and impotence.
Trade names include Navidrex

Cytotec Trade name for misoprostol

Daktarin Trade name for miconazole

Danazol

Drug which is often used in the treatment of breast pain and endometriosis, a common gynaecological disorder. Works by counteracting the natural female hormone estrogen.

Common side-effects include nausea, giddiness, weight gain, backache, rash, flushes, reduced breast size, spots, deeper voice.
Trade names include Danol

Danol *see danazol*

Decortisyl Trade name for prednisone

De-Nol, De-Noltab Trade name for bismuth chelate

Dextropropoxyphene

Pain-killer, related to morphine but milder. Carries some risk of addiction and must be used with caution. On no account exceed the stated dose. Possible side-effects may include sickness,

dizziness, drowsiness, constipation.
Trade names include Doloxene

DF118 Trade name for dihydrocodeine

DHC Continus Trade name for dihydrccodeine

Diabinese *see* ***chlorpropamide***

Diazepam

Tranquilliser which was prescribed, under the
trade name Valium, on a truly massive scale
across the globe during the 1970s and 1980s,
and is still much used today. Works by damping
down brain activity, thereby lessening anxiety.

Unfortunately, this tranquilliser can also
produce drowsiness and light-headedness which
may interfere with driving and other complex
tasks. Furthermore, most people will become
habituated ('hooked') in a very short time, so
these days diazepam should not normally be
prescribed for more than two to four weeks.
Trade names include Valium, Diazemuls, Stesolid,
Valrelease, Zetran

Diclofenac

Anti-rheumatic and pain-reliever. Diclofenac is one
of the 'non-steroidal anti-inflammatory drugs'
(see **NSAIDS** in **Classes of Drugs** for mode of
action and side-effects). This drug is mainly used
in treating arthritis of various kinds and gout, and
also in relieving pain after operations.

Do not take it if you have had ulcers, as it can
make these flare up. Diclofenac can also cause
skin reactions.
Trade names include Voltarol, Volraman, Voltaren

Digitoxin   Very similar to digoxin *(see below)*

Digoxin

Drug which helps the heart. This enormously useful agent is a 'descendant' of digitalis, the old remedy extracted from foxglove. It is used in heart failure and in treating certain abnormal heart rhythms, particularly one called atrial fibrillation. It mainly works by increasing the power of the heartbeat and by affecting the way in which electrical impulses spread through it.

Possible side-effects include nausea, diarrhoea, eyesight disturbances and an excessively slow pulse rate.

Trade names include Lanoxin, Lanoxicaps

Dihydrocodeine

Agent useful against moderate to severe pain. A milder relative of morphine. Dihydrocodeine must not be taken with alcohol.

Possible side-effects include excessive sedation, headache and dizziness.

Trade names include DF118 Forte, DHC Continus

Diltiazem

This drug is used against angina and high blood pressure. One of the group described as 'calcium antagonists' (see **calcium antagonists** in **Classes of Drugs**).

Possible side-effects include ankle swelling, nausea, flushes, tummy upsets and heartbeat abnormalities.

Trade names include Adizem, Britiazim, Dilzem, Tildiem, Cardizem

Dilzem   Trade name for diltiazem

Dimotane Trade name for brompheniramine

Dirythmin SA Trade name for disopyramide

Disipal Trade name for orphenadrine

Disopyramide
Drug which corrects abnormal heart rhythms.
Does this by slowing the rate at which nerve
impulses flow through the heart.

Possible side-effects include constipation, dry
mouth, blurred vision, low blood pressure, and
attacks of low blood sugar.
Trade names include Rythmodan, Dirythmin SA,
Napamide, Norpace, Norpace CR

Disprol paediatric Trade name for
paracetamol

Distaclor Trade name for cefaclor

Disulfiram
Drug intended to combat alcohol abuse. The
patient takes it of his own volition, knowing that
if he drinks alcohol while he is on it, the
combination of the two will give him a violent
and extremely unpleasant reaction, with nausea
and flushing. Disulfiram may help some alcohol
dependents to give up drinking.

Possible side-effects include tiredness,
bad breath, reduced sex drive.
Trade names include Antabuse

Dothiepin
Drug used against depression (see **anti-
depressants** in **Classes of Drugs** for mode of

action and possible side-effects). Dothiepin is fairly sedative compared with other anti-depressants, which may be a positive factor if you are very anxious or find it hard to sleep.
Trade names include Prothiaden

Doxepin
Drug used in depression (*see **anti-depressants** under **Classes of Drugs** for mode of action and possible side-effects.*) Like dothiepin (*see above*) doxepin is rather sedative, so it can make you feel calm or drowsy.
Trade names include Sinequan, Adapin

Doxycycline
Antibiotic (s*ee **antibiotics** under **Classes of Drugs**).* Doxycycline is effective against a wide range of germs, and is useful in treating sinusitis and other respiratory infections, chronic bronchitis, and acne (long-term use only in the case of acne). It must be taken with food.

Possible side-effects include stomach upsets, allergic reactions, and colitis.
Trade names include Vibramycin, Nordox, Doryx, Doxy-Caps, Vibra-Tabs

Dozic Trade name for haloperidol

Duphalac Trade name for lactulose

Dydrogesterone
Multi-purpose gynaecological drug, used to treat period pain, heavy menstrual bleeding, pre-menstrual syndrome (PMS), endometriosis, some cases of infertility and also sometimes menopausal symptoms. Works because it mimics the effect of the natural female hormone called

progesterone. Possible side-effects include bleeding from the vagina, which is usually an indication to increase the dose, if your doctor will agree to do so.

For further advice about side-effects, consult your GP or gynaecologist.

Trade names include Duphaston

Dyspamet Trade name for cimetidine

Elantan Trade name for isosorbide mononitrate

Emcor Trade name for bisoprolol

Enalapril

Drug used to treat heart failure and raised blood pressure. *(see **ACE-inhibitors** in **Classes of Drugs**).* Takes effect within about 90 minutes.

Possible side-effects include excessively low blood pressure, kidney problems, skin eruptions, headache, tiredness and cough.

Trade names include Innovace, Vasotec

Ephedrine

Old-fashioned drug, but still useful in relieving various conditions, notably nasal congestion as a cold symptom, asthma and other forms of obstruction of the airways, although more modern drugs are generally used these days. (It is also used for diabetic nerve damage, and occasionally bed-wetting in older children.)

It mainly works by shrinking up inflamed tissues and widening the airways.

WARNING: do not take ephedrine before any sports competition; in most sports it is banned

because of its stimulant effect.
Possible side-effects include excessive brain
stimulation, anxiety, sleeplessness, trembling.
Trade names include CAM

Erymax, Erythrocin, Erythromid, Erythroped, Eramycin
Trade names for erythromycin (see below)

Erythromycin
Widely-prescribed antibiotic (see **antibiotics** under
Classes of Drugs). Works by stopping bacteria
from breeding. Useful for ear and respiratory
infections, whooping cough, some internal pelvic
infections in women and also legionnaire's
disease. An excellent alternative to penicillin for
the many people who are allergic to it. Usually
taken on an empty stomach ask your doctor.

Possible side-effects include sickness, tummy
discomfort, diarrhoea, rashes and occasionally
jaundice (yellowness).
Among an enormous number of possible trade
names are Erymax, Erythrocin, Erythromid,
Erythroped (mainly for children), Ilosone, EES,
E-Mycin, Eramycin, Ethril, Wyamycin

Etidronate
Treatment for Paget's disease and osteoporosis,
the 'thinning bones' condition common after the
age of 45. Stops calcium leaking from the bones.

Possible side-effects include sickness, diarrhoea,
and an odd taste in the mouth.
Trade names include Didronel, Didronel PMO (a
combination with calcium)

Fenbufen
Non-steroidal anti-inflammatory drug (see **NSAIDs**

*in **Classes of Drugs**)*. Used in treating various kinds of arthritis and rheumatism. Works by damping down inflammation.

Possible side-effects can include rashes, in which case discontinue use, tummy upsets, and – more rarely – allergic lung problems.
Do not take Fenbufen if you have an ulcer.
Trade names include Lederfen

Fersaday, Fergon, Ferromyn, Fer-In-Sol, Fer Iron, Ferospace
Trade names for iron preparations (*see below*)

Ferrous fumarate, ferrous gluconate, ferrous succinate, ferrous sulphate
These are all iron preparations, used to treat the very common condition of iron-deficiency anaemia (weak blood). All of them are effective in getting the blood count back to normal over a period of time. Though these preparations are best absorbed if taken on an empty stomach, they may have to be taken after meals to avoid stomach upsets.

Possible side-effects include stomach ache, nausea and diarrhoea, or constipation. Bowel motions may turn black, but this does not matter.
Trade names: there are many brand names worldwide, mostly beginning with the letters 'Fer-'

Finasteride
A relatively new drug, used to treat enlargement of the prostate gland. Works by blocking the manufacture of a form of male hormone.

Possible side-effects include lowered sexual desire, impotence, and decreased volume of seminal fluid.

Trade names include Proscar

Flagyl Trade name for metronidazole

Flemoxin Trade name for amoxycillin

Flucloxacillin
Antibiotic *(see **antibiotics** under **Classes of Drugs**)*. Used mainly for infections which are resistant to penicillin. Possible side-effects include those of penicillin, plus jaundice
Trade names include Floxapen, Stafoxil

Fluconazole
Anti-fungal drug, used mainly to treat vaginal thrush. Unlike most other thrush preparations, it is not given via the vagina, but taken by mouth. Some women prefer this as it is less messy

Possible side-effects include nausea, wind, diarrhoea, tummy ache and skin problems. It must not be taken if you are on certain hay fever remedies. Further advice will be available from your doctor or pharmacist.
Trade names include Diflucan

Fluoxetine
Anti-depressant which has become famous worldwide in the 1990s, under the trade name Prozac. Controversy has pursued this drug, but early newspaper reports that it has caused suicide have not been substantiated.

Fluoxetine is not chemically related to the older drugs for depression *(see **anti-depressants** under **Classes of Drugs**)*. It appears to work by helping a natural brain chemical called serotonin to enter nerve cells. This seems to help improve mood and alertness and may return sleep patterns to normal. It is important to realise that the drug takes several weeks to produce an anti-depressant effect and that it will stay in your body for some time after you stop it.

Possible side-effects include impairment of driving and other complex tasks, skin problems, allergic reactions, anxiety, drowsiness, trembling, sweating, insomnia, dry mouth, throat and lung inflammation, sexual malfunction, convulsions and anorexia with weight loss.
Trade names include Prozac

Flurbiprofen
Non-steroidal anti-inflammatory drug *(see **NSAIDs** under **Classes of Drugs**)*, used against arthritis and rheumatism. Should be taken after food.

Possible side-effects include tummy upsets, abdominal pain, rash and jaundice (yellowness). Do not take if you have had ulcers.
Trade names include Froben, Ansaid

Folic Acid
Important member of the B group of vitamins. Essential for life, as it is needed by the body for cell growth. Lack of it leads eventually to an unusual and severe type of anaemia. Fortunately, the average Western diet contains enough leafy green vegetables to provide adequate amounts. But recent research strongly suggests that women who are in early pregnancy and those trying for a baby should take 0.4 milligrammes daily in order to try to reduce the risk of spina bifida.

In many countries, a small dose of folic acid, combined with iron, is given throughout the term

of a pregnancy in order to prevent anaemia. Side-effects are rare, but this vitamin should never be taken in cases of anaemia or cancer unless a doctor has confirmed that it is the appropriate treatment.
Trade names include Lexpec

Frusemide, Furosemide
'Water tablet' or diuretic (see **diuretics** in **Classes of Drugs**). Used to treat oedema (dropsy), heart failure, and raised blood pressure. Works by inducing the kidney to pass more urine.

Possible side-effects include gout, rashes, tummy upsets, disturbances in blood minerals.
Trade names include Lasix

Furadantin Trade name for nitrofurantoin

Furosemide Alternative name for frusemide
(see above)

Fusidic acid
Antibiotic (see **antibiotics** under **Classes of Drugs**). Used against penicillin-resistant staphylococcal infections.

Side-effects include sickness, rashes and liver problems. Indeed, patients who are on this drug should have regular blood tests to check liver function.
Trade names include Fucidin

GTN see glyceryl trinitrate

Galenamet Trade name for cimetidine

Galenamox Trade name for amoxycillin

Galpseud Trade name for pseudoephedrine

Gamolenic acid

An extract of evening primrose, used to treat eczema and persistent breast pain. Gamolenic acid has not long been used by orthodox medicine, and a good deal remains to be discovered about its affects and possible uses.

Possible side-effects include nausea, headache and possibly exacerbation of epilepsy. Please note that in breast pain, the drug takes several months to produce an effect.
Trade names include Efamast, Epogam

Gastrobid Continus, Gastromax

Trade names for metoclopramide, in sustained release form

Gentamicin

Antibiotic (*see* **antibiotics** *under* **Classes of Drugs**).

Used to cure eye and ear infections. Also used against certain overwhelming infections, such as septicaemia (blood poisoning).

Side-effects are uncommon when the drug is used for eye and ear infections, but when it is administered to treat much more severe infections, it can cause damage to hearing, to balance mechanisms and to the kidneys.

Glibenclamide

Drug used to treat the type of diabetes which does not require insulin injections. Must be combined with a strict diet. Works mainly by increasing a person's own production of insulin.

Side-effects include sensitivity rashes, occasional blood problems, and – very importantly – low blood sugar attacks. Best avoided in elderly people because of the risk of these attacks.
Trade names include Daonil, Euglucon, Semi-Daonil

Gliclazide
Anti-diabetes drug. Similar in many ways to glibenclamide (*see above*), but can usually be used in the elderly.
Trade names include Diamicron

Glyceryl trinitrate
Long-established, but still very useful drug used in preventing and relieving attacks of angina. Traditionally, it is taken under the tongue – if possible, just before a slight exertion. A tablet or spray may be used, but these days it can also be given via a skin patch, or even as an ointment. 'GTN' works mainly by reducing the work load on the heart.

Possible side-effects include throbbing headache, flushes, giddiness and fainting.
Trade names: worldwide there are many dozens of brand names for this popular drug. Among the best known are: Coro-Nitro Spray, Glytrin Spray, Nitrolingual Spray, Suscard, Sustac, Percutol, Deponit, Minitran, Nitro-Dur, Transderm-Nitro, Nitrogard, Nitroglyn, Nitrolin, Nitronet, Nitrong, Nitrospan, Nitrostat

Goserelin
One of a relatively new group of drugs (the 'GnRH analogues') which are being used to treat the common gynaecological condition called endometriosis, and also sometimes breast and prostate cancer. They work by lowering blood

levels of the female hormone oestrogen. In males, they lower the levels of male hormone.

Side-effects include menopause-type symptoms, such as hot flushes and vaginal dryness, and also headaches, reduced breast size and reduced sex drive.

Griseofulvin

Anti-fungus drug, widely used against fungal infection of the skin, scalp and nails, where treatment with ointments has persistently failed. Works because it is good at 'lodging' itself in the keratin of skin and nails. Has to be taken for several months for effects to take place.

Side-effects include sickness, headache, rashes, light sensitivity.
Trade names include Fulcin, Grisovin

Haldol Trade name for haloperidol (*see below*)

Haloperidol

Extremely powerful tranquilliser, used in the treatment of serious illnesses, such as schizophrenia. Works by blocking 'nerve transmitters' in the brain. It is also used to treat intractable hiccups.

Possible side-effects include drowsiness and odd movements of the muscles, particularly of the face and tongue.
Trade names include Haldol, Dozic

Hamarin Trade name for allopurinol

Hismanal Trade name for astemizole

Hydralazine

Drug used against heart failure and high blood pressure. Works by widening blood vessels. Side-effects include faint feelings, flushes, headaches, joint pain, angina and – very importantly – development of systemic lupus, a connective tissue disease.
Trade names include Apresoline

Hydroxychloroquine

Drug used against rheumatoid arthritis and also systemic lupus, a connective tissue disease.

Possible side-effects include eye damage, skin reactions, bleaching of the hair and bald patches.
Trade names include Plaquenil

Hypovase Trade name for prazosin

Ibuprofen

A non-steroidal anti-inflammatory drug *(see **NSAIDs** under **Classes of Drugs**)*, used in treating arthritis, and pain generally. In fact, it is exactly the same as the widely-used over the counter pain-killer Nurofen. Best taken after food.

Possible side-effects include stomach ache, internal bleeding, rash. Do not take if you have had an ulcer, unless your doctor feels that no other treatment is suitable for you.
Trade names include Brufen, Junifen, Motrin, Pamprin-B, Rufen

Imdur Trade name for isosorbide mononitrate

Imipramine

Anti-depressant *(see **anti-depressants** under **Classes of Drugs**)*. An old-established drug, imipramine is thought to work by prolonging the life of two brain chemicals which are probably deficient in many cases of depression. Less sedative than some other anti-depressants, so less liable to make you drowsy.

Possible side-effects include dry mouth, blurred vision, nausea, constipation.
Trade names include Tofranil, Tipramine, Janimine

Imperacin Trade name for oxytetracycline

Imtack Trade name for isosorbide dinitrate

Inderal Trade name for propranolol

Indomethacin
Non-steroidal anti-inflammatory drug *(see **NSAIDs** under **Classes of Drugs**)*, widely used to treat arthritis, gout, back pain, various rheumatic disorders, and also period pain. Take with food.

Possible side-effects are headaches, internal bleeding from the stomach, tummy upsets, eye problems, dizziness, diarrhoea. Better avoided if you have had an ulcer.

Indoramin
Drug which is used to treat (a) raised blood pressure (b) enlargement of the prostate gland. It lowers blood pressure by opening up the tubes through which the blood flows. In prostate trouble, indoramin relaxes muscles near the bladder's outlet, making it easier to pass urine.

Possible side-effects include a dry mouth, sleepiness, nasal congestion, weight gain and difficulty with male sexual climax.

Trade names include: Baratol, Doralese

Ipral Trade name for trimethoprim

Ipratropium
Anti-asthma drug. Works by relaxing, and therefore opening, the tubes which carry air into the lungs. It is slow to take effect, but gives good long-term protection against asthma attacks in some people. It can also be used against hay fever and related conditions.

Possible side-effects include dryness of the mouth and difficulty in passing urine.
Trade names include Atrovent, Rinatec

Ismo Trade name for isosorbide mononitrate

Isoket, Isordil Trade names for isosorbide dinitrate (see below)

Isosorbide dinitrate, isosorbide mononitrate
Two closely-related drugs which are used in the treatment of heart failure, and in the prevention and treatment of angina. Both drugs are very similar in action and side-effects to glyceryl trinitrate *(see **glyceryl trinitrate**)*, but they are available in formulations which have a longer-lasting effect. Among a multitude of trade names which are prescribed in various countries, the following are probably the best known:

Isosorbide dinitrate: Cedocard, Imtack, Isoket, Isordil, Dilatrate-SA, Iso-Bid, Isonate, Onset, Sorate.

Isosorbide mononitrate: Elantan, Imdur, Ismo, Isotrate, Monit, Mono-Cedocard, MCR-50

Isotrate Trade name for isosorbide mononitrate

Kay-Cee-L Trade name for potassium chloride

Keflex Trade name for cephalexin

Kemadrin Trade name for procyclidine

Ketoconazole
Anti-fungus drug, mainly used to treat women with vaginal thrush (candida, monilia). Works by attacking the cell wall of the fungus. Taken by mouth, with food, unlike many other anti-fungals which are applied directly. Do not take with Hismanal.

Possible side-effects include rashes, headaches, swollen breasts, gastric upsets, liver problems.
Trade names include Nizoral

Ketoprofen
Non-steroidal anti-inflammatory drug (see **NSAIDs in Classes of Drugs**), used to treat gout, period pain, most types of muscle and joint pain and mild inflammation. Take with food. Do not take if you have an ulcer or a history of recurrent ulcers.

Possible side-effects include gastric irritation, internal bleeding from the stomach, rashes, dizziness, headache, drowsiness.
Trade names include Alrheumat, Orudis, Oruvail

Ketotifen
Anti-allergy drug for asthma attacks, allergic conjunctivitis, allergic rhinitis such as hay fever. Side-effects include sleepiness (so avoid driving and operating machinery), giddiness, dry mouth.
Trade names include Zaditen

Klaricid Trade name for clarithromycin

Labetalol

Drug used against high blood pressure, especially where the person also has angina. It works by widening blood vessels. Best taken with food.

Possible side-effects include faintness, especially on standing up, tiredness, headaches, skin rashes, sickness, tingling on the scalp.
Trade names include Trandate, Normodyne

Lactugal Trade name for lactulose (see below)

Lactulose

Agent used for constipation. Works by retaining water inside the bowel, encouraging it to contract. Side-effects include cramps and wind.
Trade names include Duphalac, Lactugal

Lanoxin Trade name for digoxin

Largactil Trade name for chlorpromazine

Lentizol Trade name for amitriptyline

Levodopa (L-dopa)

Useful drug in Parkinson's disease. Acts mainly by replenishing the brain's stores of dopamine, a natural chemical lacking in this ailment. Speeds up movement and reduces stiffness, but less effective in reducing tremor. It is usually taken after meals for the best effect.

Possible side-effects include sickness, loss of appetite, anxiety, sleeplessness, dizziness, red discoloration of urine.
Trade names include Brocadopa, Larodopa, Dopar

Librium Trade name for chlordiazepoxide

Li-Liquid Trade name for lithium citrate

Lisinopril
Drug used in high blood pressure, and heart failure (see **ACE-inhibitors** under **Classes of Drugs**).

Possible side-effects include palpitations, faintness, rashes, headaches, kidney problems, cough, diarrhoea.
Trade names include Zestril, Carace, Prinivil

Liskonium Trade name for lithium carbonate (see below)

Litarex Trade name for lithium citrate (see **lithium** below)

Lithium
Used to treat manic-depressive illness, and also recurrent depression. Lithium is actually a metal, very like sodium, of which there is a great deal in the body. Replacing a little of the sodium with lithium tends to calm down extreme emotions such as excitement and misery.

Do not take lithium with hot drinks. Blood levels of the metal must be checked from time to time.

Possible side-effects include stomach upsets, thirst, passing a lot of urine and tremor.
Trade names include Camcolit, Priadel, Li-Liquid, Liskonium, Litarex, Cibalith-S, Eskalith, Lithane, Lithobid, Lithonate, Lithotabs

Loperamide

Anti-diarrhoeal. Works by damping down the nerves which supply the bowel. Should only be given when the cause of the diarrhoea is known – it treats only the symptom, not the cause.

Possible side-effects include rashes, cramps, dry mouth.
Trade names include Imodium, Loperagen, Imodium-AD

Lopresor Trade name for metoprolol

Lorazepam

Strong tranquilliser which gained fame and much media exposure in the 1980s, under the brand name Ativan. Acts by damping down brain activity. Unfortunately, lorazepam tends to make people 'hooked' quite rapidly, so these days most doctors will only prescribe it for very short periods.

Possible side-effects include drowsiness, depression, habituation, and withdrawal symptoms if the drug is stopped suddenly.
Trade names include Ativan, Alzapam

Macrobid, Macrodantin Trade names for nitrofurantoin

Magnesium hydroxide and magnesium sulphate (Epsom salts)

Traditional drugs used as laxatives. Work by 'pulling' water into the bowel, which encourages it to contract. Both drugs are often grossly over-used by the public; in general it is best to take them only on medical advice.

Possible side-effects include 'numbing' and loss of bowel function after long-term use.

Maxolon Trade name for metoclopramide

MCR-50 Trade name for isosorbide mononitrate

Mebeverine
Anti-spasmodic drug, used to relieve intestinal spasm and irritable bowel syndrome. Believed to work by relaxing muscle in the gut wall.
Trade names include: Colofac

Mefenamic acid
Non-steroidal anti-inflammatory drug *(see **NSAIDs** in **Classes of Drugs**)*, much used in arthritis, rheumatic conditions and muscle/joint pain – and, increasingly these days, in period pain. Also of use in reducing heavy menstrual flow. Best taken after food. Do not take if you have ulcers or inflammatory bowel disease.

Side-effects include stomach ache, stomach upsets, rashes, drowsiness.
Trade names include Ponstan, Ponstan Forte

Melleril Trade name for thioridazine

Metformin
Anti-diabetic drug, used in diabetics who do not need insulin injections. Must be combined with a strict diet. Works by various mechanisms which lower blood sugar.

Possible side-effects include excessively low blood sugar, loss of appetite, sickness and/or diarrhoea.
Trade names include: Glucophage

Methadone

Drug from the morphine 'family', used for (a) severe pain, (b) suppressing cough in terminal illness, (c) trying to wean addicts off even stronger drugs.

Side-effects include addiction, sickness, constipation, drowsiness.
Trade names include Physeptone

Methimazole

'Anti-thyroid' drug, very similar to neo-mercazole *(please see **neo-mercazole**)*.

Methyldopa

Drug for high blood pressure. Acts by widening blood vessels, the tubes which carry blood.

Side-effects include sleepiness, headache, depression, stuffy nose, dry mouth, problems with male sexual climax, significant blood changes. Do not drive while on this drug.
Trade names include Aldomet

Methysergide

Drug used to try to prevent migraine attacks. Works by altering brain chemicals. Best taken with meals.

Possible side-effects include nausea, tummy discomfort, tiredness, cramps, hair loss and – most importantly, though rarely – internal 'fibrosis' (thickening in the membranes inside the body).
Trade names include Deseril

Metoclopramide

Drug used against dyspepsia and nausea. Works by means of several complex actions on the gut, stomach and brain. Best avoided in the under-20s, except in cases of intractable vomiting, because of the risk of causing severe muscle spasms in the face.

Other possible side-effects include drowsiness, restlessness, depression, diarrhoea.
Trade names include Maxolon, Gastrobid Continus, Gastromax, Clopra, Octamide, Reclomide, Reglan

Metoprolol
Beta-blocker drug (*see **beta-blockers** in **Classes of Drugs***), used to treat high blood pressure, angina, irregular heart rhythms and also to try and prevent migraine attacks.

Metoprolol is a 'heart-selective' beta-blocker, and so is less likely to cause unwanted effects elsewhere in the body. Nonetheless, possible side-effects include tiredness, wheeze, cold hands and feet, and tummy upsets.
Trade names include Betaloc, Lopresor

Metronidazole
Drug which is effective against various disease-producing micro-organisms, but in particular *Trichomonas vaginalis*, which is a common cause of vaginal discharge. Metronidazole is also useful against mouth infections caused by the same organism, and against certain tropical infections.

Possible side-effects include sickness, unpleasant taste and rashes. Do not take alcohol while on this drug, as the combination may cause collapse.
Trade names include Flagyl, Zadstat, Femazole, Metizol, Protostat

Mianserin

Anti-depressant *(see **anti-depressants** under **Classes of Drugs**)*. Its method of action is not yet completely understood, but it usually lifts the mood within a fortnight or so.

Possible side-effects include sleepiness, jaundice (yellowness), joint pain and blood problems – most doctors will do regular blood tests while you are on it.

Trade names include Bolvidon, Norval

Miconazole

Anti-fungus drug, widely used for infections of the mouth, the skin and the vagina. Works by attacking the cell wall of the fungus.

When taken by mouth, it can cause tummy upsets. Some people are allergic to application to skin, and may develop redness and itching.

Trade names include Daktarin, Micatin, Monistat-3, Monistat-7, Monistat-Derm

Minoxidil

Anti-blood pressure drug which attained media fame in the 1980s as the world's first genuine hair-restorer under the trade names Regaine and Rogaine. In high blood pressure, minoxidil – taken by mouth – works by widening the blood vessels.

Side-effects of this method of treatment include oedema (dropsy), rapid heart beat, and occasionally excessive hair growth.

For baldness, the drug is applied as a solution to the scalp, twice daily. Some men (unfortunately, very far from all) get an appreciable regrowth of hair, or at least a cessation of hair loss.

Possible side-effects include scalp irritation.
Trade names for the blood pressure version of
the drug include Loniten

Misoprostol
Anti-ulcer drug, used particularly for treating or
trying to prevent stomach ulcers caused by
pain-killers *(see **NSAIDs** under **Classes of Drugs)**.*
Works in various ways, including increasing the
protective mucous lining of the stomach.

Possible side-effects include diarrhoea, stomach
ache, period problems, rash.
Trade names include Cytotec

Monit, Mono-Cedocard Trade names for
isosorbide mononitrate

Monocor Trade name for bisoprolol

Motilium Trade name for domperidone

Morphine
Very powerful pain-killer, unfortunately with an
enormous capacity for causing addiction, so
it is only used sparingly, in cases of great pain.
Believed to work by mimicking the action of
certain natural pain-killers inside the brain.
Side-effects include addiction, nausea, vomiting,
drowsiness, constipation, breathing difficulties.
Trade names include Oramorph, Sevredol, MST
Continus, SRM-Rhotard

Mysoline Trade name for primidone

Nafarelin
Nasal spray, used to treat the common
gynaecological condition endometriosis and also

a few cases of female infertility, prior to IVF therapy. Works by affecting the way in which the pituitary gland stimulates the ovaries.

Possible side-effects include vaginal bleeding, menopause-type symptoms, loss of sex drive, thin bones, smaller breasts.

Do not use at same time as any kind of nasal decongestant spray.
Trade names include Synarel

Naprosyn Trade name for naproxen (*see below*)

Naproxen
Non-steroidal anti-inflammatory drug *(see **NSAIDs** under **Classes of Drugs**)*, much used in arthritis and gout, and for the relief of pain, including period pain. Do not take if you have an ulcer.

Possible side-effects include stomach irritation, internal bleeding, rash, headache, ringing in the ears.
Trade names include Naprosyn, Nycopren, Synflex, Anaprox

Neo-Mercazole Trade name for carbimazole

Nicardipine
Drug used in the treatment of angina and high blood pressure. *(see **calcium antagonists** in **Classes of Drugs** for mode of action)*. Best taken on an empty stomach.

Possible side-effects include heart pain, in which case the drug must be stopped, headache, giddiness, 'flushed' sensations, oedema (dropsy).
Trade names include Cardene

Nifedipine

Used in angina, high blood pressure, and Raynaud's phenomenon, a constriction of the blood vessels in the fingers *(see **calcium antagonists** in **Classes of Drugs** for mode of action)*.

Possible side-effects include heart pain – in which case stop taking the medication – headache, flushing, giddiness, tiredness, oedema (dropsy), diarrhoea.
Trade names include Adalat, Coracten, Nimotop

Nitrofurantoin

Drug used against urinary infections, such as cystitis and pyelitis. Always try to send your urine specimen to the lab before starting the drug, otherwise it may make the test invalid. Best taken with food.

Possible side-effects include loss of appetite, nausea, tummy upset.
Trade names include Furadantin, Macrobid, Macrodantin, Furan, Furalan, Furanite, Nitrofan

Nitroglycerin *see glyceryl trinitrate*

Nivaquine Trade name for chloroquine

Normison Trade name for temazepam

Noctec Trade name for chloral

Nortriptyline

Anti-depressant *(see **anti-depressants** under **Classes of Drugs**.* Works mainly by prolonging the effect of two natural 'mood lifting' chemicals in the brain. May well take a fortnight to have effect. Nortriptyline is less sedative than some other anti-depressants.

Possible side-effects may include dry mouth, constipation, blurry vision, sickness, difficulty in passing water.
Trade names include Aventyl, Allegron, Pamelor

Norval Trade name for mianserin

Nycopren Trade name for naproxen

Nystan Trade name for nystatin (*see below*)

Nystatin
Anti-fungal drug used against thrush (monilia, candida) in the vagina, on the skin, in the mouth and round the anus.

When applied directly to the vagina, skin, mouth or anus, nystatin is very unlikely to produce side-effects, though it will stain clothes yellow. Oral tablets of nystatin can sometimes produce sickness, diarrhoea and rashes.
Trade names include Nystan, Mycostatin, Nilstat

Nuelin Trade name for theophylline

Omeprazole
Widely used against gastric (stomach) and duodenal ulcers, and for oesophagitis (inflammation of the gullet). Works by blocking the mechanisms which produce stomach acid.

Possible side-effects include copious diarrhoea, severe headache, sickness, constipation, wind, sleepiness and dizziness.
Trade names include Losec

Orciprenaline

Anti-asthma drug, also useful in chronic bronchitis and emphysema. Works by widening air passages. Available as aerosol, syrup and tablets.

Possible side-effects include tremor, nerviness, headache, heart irregularities.
Trade names include Alupent

Orphenadrine

Drug for Parkinsonism. Works by helping to correct a chemical imbalance in the brain. Reduces tremors and rigidity to some extent, but not as effective as levodopa *(see **levodopa**)*, with which it is often combined. Can reduce dribbling.

Possible side effects include insomnia, dry mouth, giddiness, blurred vision, tummy upsets.
Trade names include Disipal, Biorphen

Oxprenolol

Drug used for high blood pressure, angina, irregularities of heartbeat, and also sometimes for anxiety. *(Please see **beta-blockers** under **Classes of Drugs**)*. Take with food if it upsets your stomach.

Possible side-effects include sickness, dizziness, tingling in the scalp, distortion of taste, tiredness, sweating and impotence.
Trade names include Trasicor, Slow-Trasicor

Oxytetracycline

Antibiotic *(see **tetracyclines** under the heading **antibiotics** in **Classes of Drugs**)*. Useful in chronic bronchitis and certain pelvic infections in women. Also taken long-term for acne treatment.

Possible side-effects include diarrhoea, sickness, thrush, or a red rash on the skin (stop taking if this occurs).
Trade names include Terramycin, Imperacin

Paldesic, Panadol, Panaleve
Trade names for paracetamol (see below)

Paracetamol (known in much of the world as acetaminophen)
Very useful pain-killer; also lowers fever. Particularly useful nowadays for children, since they should not have aspirin (*see aspirin).* Paracetamol is much less irritant to the stomach than aspirin and other widely-used pain-killers. But accidental over-dosage can easily happen, and may prove fatal – even though the person appears well for some days. So at all costs, do not exceed the correct dose for the patient's age or weight.

Side-effects include liver damage, rashes, blood problems, inflammation of the pancreas.
Among a multitude of trade names world-wide are Calpol, Panadol, Cupanol, Disprol Paediatric, Paldesic, Panaleve, Salzone, Tylenol, Actamin, Tempra

Paroxetine
Anti-depressant *(see **anti-depressants** under **Classes of Drugs**)*. Works by increasing the amount of a natural brain chemical called '5HT'. Useful in depression accompanied by anxiety.

Possible side-effects include sedation – so it may affect driving and other complex skills – sickness, sweating, tremor, dry mouth, fits, sex difficulties.
Trade names include Seroxat

Pecram Trade name for aminophylline

Penbritin Trade name for ampicillin

Penicillin
The first ever antibiotic, and a very useful one
*(see **penicillins** under the heading **antibiotics** in*
***Classes of Drugs**).*

There are many different varieties of penicillin,
but they are all useful against bacteria which
often cause such conditions as sore throat, ear
ache, skin infections and pneumonia. However,
penicillin has absolutely no effect on viruses,
including the ones that cause colds. Also,
penicillin-resistant strains of bacteria have
emerged in the last few decades. Taking penicillin
for trivial things encourages the emergence of
such resistance.

The most frequent side-effect of penicillin is
allergy (hypersensitivity), which usually causes a
distressingly itchy rash. However, hypersensitivity
to penicillin occasionally causes potentially fatal
collapse. If you are sensitive to penicillin, make
sure that you always carry a written warning next
to your I.D. Similarly, your records at your family
doctor's and/or hospital should be clearly marked
'penicillin sensitive' on the cover.

Pentazocine
Powerful pain-killer of the morphine group,
although not as strong, and with much less risk
of addiction. Works by mimicking natural
pain-killers produced in the brain. Do not drink
alcohol while on this drug.

Possible side-effects include sleepiness, poor
co-ordination, sickness, constipation, and

occasionally hallucinations.
Trade names include Fortral and also Talwin NX,
a special formulation designed to prevent abuse

Phenergan   Trade name for promethazine

Phyllocontin   Trade name for aminophylline

Piriton   Trade name for chlorpheniramine

Piroxicam
Non-steroidal anti-inflammatory drug *(see **NSAIDs**
under **Classes of Drugs**)*. Piroxicam is widely
used for the relief of pain and inflammation,
particularly in arthritis and gout. It is best taken
with food.

Possible side-effects include stomach upsets and
pain, allergy, blood problems, inflammation of the
pancreas, blurred vision.
Trade names include Feldene

Pizotifen
Anti-migraine drug, used for prevention – rather
than treatment – of attacks. Its method of action
isn't yet entirely clear.

Possible side-effects include weight gain and
drowsiness, so avoid driving and complex tasks.
Trade names include Sanomigran

Potassium chloride, KCl
Mineral replacement. A lot of people need to take
potassium chloride because of the fact that their
bodies' potassium stores have been lowered by
the effect of 'water pills' *(see **diuretics** under
Classes of Drugs)*. There are also other
circumstances where taking potassium chloride in

the exact amounts prescribed by your doctor may be – literally – life-saving.

Possible side-effects of KCl, as potassium chloride is sometimes known, include nausea, vomiting, and ulceration in the gullet or intestine. Tell your doctor if you develop any digestive problems at all.
Trade names include Kay-Cee-L, Slow-K, Kay Ciel, Klor, K-Tab

Prazosin

A drug for lowering high blood pressure. Prazosin is also used in heart failure and Raynaud's disease, and sometimes for urinary retention. Works by a relaxation effect, which opens up the blood vessels.

Unfortunately, the first dose may do this quite dramatically and cause a faint, so it is best taken at bedtime. Other possible side-effects include drowsiness, headache, sickness, palpitations.
Trade names include Hypovase, Minipress

Precortisyl (Forte), Prednesol Trade
names for prednisolone (*see below*)

Prednisolone

Powerful steroid drug *(see **steroids** under **Classes of Drugs**).*

Prednisolone is in effect a successor of the famous cortisone, which created such a sensation when it was first used 50 years ago. Prednisolone has a very strong anti-inflammatory effect, which makes it very useful in a wide variety of ailments, including severe asthma, serious inflammatory and allergic skin diseases, rheumatoid arthritis (not 'ordinary'

arthritis', in which case it may be harmful),
ulcerative colitis, Crohn's disease, gout and many
other conditions.

It can have extremely serious side-effects, so it is
VITAL to stick precisely to the dose your doctor
has prescribed, and not to take the drug for
longer than absolutely necessary. At the end of a
course, it must be 'tailed off' gradually. Possible
side-effects include growth stunting in children,
moderately raised blood pressure, ulcers,
diabetes, osteoporosis (thin bones), and flare-ups
of infection.
Trade names include Prednesol, Precortisyl
(Forte)

Prednisone
Powerful steroid drug; very similar to
prednisolone *(see above)*.
Trade names include Decortisyl, Deltasone,
Orasone, Sterapred

Pro-Actidil Trade name for triprolidine

Priadel Trade name for lithium carbonate

Primidone
Anti-epilepsy drug, also sometimes used in trying
to control tremor of the hands. Works by damping
down electrical activity in the brain.

Possible side-effects include sleepiness, nausea,
incoordination, rashes and eye disturbances.
Trade names include Mysoline, Primoline

Prochlorperazine
Anti-nausea drug and powerful tranquilliser. Used
in severe nausea, and also serious mental

disturbances. Works by powerful sedative effect on the brain, and particularly on the nerve centres of the brain which cause vomiting.

Possible side-effects include deep drowsiness, and odd reactions of the muscles of the face and tongue.

Trade names include Stemetil, Buccastem, Compazine

Procyclidine
Drug for Parkinson's disease. Works by helping to correct the chemical imbalance which occurs in the brains of people with this condition.

Side-effects include dry mouth, blurred vision, stomach upsets, giddiness.

Proguanil
Anti-malarial drug, famous world-wide under the trade name of Paludrine. Taken as a protective, it should be started a week before going to the tropics and continued for four weeks after leaving. Best taken with food. Your doctor will probably advise that you take chloroquine *(see **chloroquine**)* as well.

As a result of the increasing problem of resistance to drugs, proguanil is now only effective in certain areas of the world. Obtain details from your physician or travel clinic.

Side-effects include stomach upsets, rashes, sore mouth, hair loss.

Promazine
Powerful tranquilliser, used in severe mental disturbances. Works by sedating the brain.

Possible side-effects include excessive sedation, coldness, odd reactions of the muscles of the face and tongue.
Trade names include Sparine

Promethazine
Antihistamine *(see **antihistamines** under **Classes of Drugs**)*, much used in hay fever and allergies generally, to avoid travel sickness and occasionally as a night-time sedative.

Its major drawback is that it makes people drowsy and slows reactions – driving is best avoided. Other possible side-effects include light-sensitivity reactions in the skin, and occasionally odd effects on muscle co-ordination.
Trade names include Phenergan, Avomine, Sominex

Propantheline
Used for treating ulcers and irritable bowel syndrome, and occasionally for bed-wetting. Works mainly by blocking nerves which supply the stomach and intestine.
Side-effects include blurry vision, dry mouth, difficulty in passing water.
Trade names include Pro-Banthine, Norpanth

Propranolol
One of the earliest of the famous beta-blocker group of drugs *(see **beta-blockers** under **Classes of Drugs**)*.

Used in high blood pressure, angina, disorders of heart rhythm, and also to treat the symptoms of anxiety. Some sportsmen take it for this last purpose, particularly in events where they need a steady hand, but its use could well be banned by your sport's governing body.

Possible side-effects include wheezing, sedation, slow pulse, cold hands and feet, tiredness, sleep problems, depression and heart failure.
Trade names include Inderal, Beta Prograne

Prozac Trade name for fluoxetine

Proventil Trade name for salbutamol

Pseudoephedrine
Drug used to try to relieve congestion around the nose and sinuses. Often combined with other agents in cold and cough remedies.

Warning: this drug is a stimulant, and is banned by many sporting bodies; athletes quite often get themselves into trouble by using it for presumably innocent reasons.

Side-effects may include excessive stimulation of the brain and hence restlessness and insomnia, and/or an increase in blood pressure.
Trade names include Sudafed, Galpseud, Sudrin

Pyridoxine *see **vitamin B6***

Questran Trade name for cholestyramine

Quinine
Traditional remedy for one type of malaria; much more often used in Western countries as a treatment for night-time cramps. However, deaths have occurred from overdosage, particularly in children. Do not leave lying around!

Possible ill-effects, of which there are many, include headache, ringing in the ears, sickness, tummy-ache, rashes, flushing, eye problems, feelings of confusion.

Ranitidine

Anti-ulcer drug which became famous in the 1980s and 1990s under the trade name Zantac. One of the world's most widely-used drugs, ranitidine is like cimetidine *(see **cimetidine**)* in the way it blocks acid production in the stomach.

Useful for gastric and duodenal ulcers, and also reflux oesophagitis (inflammation of the gullet). Usually taken in a short course – four to eight weeks. There are two alternative ways of taking it: either twice-daily dosage, or a single, larger dose at night.

Possible side-effects include headache, giddiness, changes in bowel habits, such as looser or less frequent motions, and occasionally confusion, swelling and tenderness of male breasts, blood or liver problems.
Trade names include Zantac

Rastinon Trade name for tolbutamide

Regaine, Rogaine Trade names for minoxidil

Rheumox Trade name for azapropazone

Rivotril Trade name for clonazepam

Rythmodan Trade name for disopyramide

Salamol Trade name for salbutamol *(see below)*

Salbulin Trade name for salbutamol *(see below)*

Salbutamol

Anti-asthma drug, also useful in other conditions
in which the 'airways' are too narrow such
as chronic bronchitis. Works by widening the
air tubes.

Salbutamol comes in various forms: tablets,
aerosols, inhaled powders, nebulised solutions
and injections. Your own physician must
determine which type is best for you. Do not
take more often than your doctor advises.

Possible side-effects include trembling of the
hands, headache, anxiety, low blood potassium,
rapid heartbeat, and hypersensitivity reactions.
Trade names include Ventolin, Volmax, Salbulin,
Salamol, Aerolin Autohaler, Ventodisks

Salmeterol

Drug used in airways obstruction (including
asthma) in patients requiring long-term treatment.
It is not intended for treating actual attacks of
asthma. Salmeterol is usually employed along
with other drugs, not on its own.

Possible side-effects include an odd reaction in
which breathing gets more difficult, instead of
easier, in which case the doctor should be
contacted at once; also headache, tremor,
palpitations, low blood potassium, cramps.
Trade names include Serevent

Selzone Trade name for paracetamol

Sanomigran Trade name for pizotifen

Sectral Trade name for acebutolol

Securon Trade name for verapamil

Selegiline
Drug for Parkinson's disease. Works by keeping up the level of a brain chemical, dopamine, which is usually deficient in Parkinsonism. Reports suggest that it can delay the disease's progress.

Possible side-effects include faintness on standing up, sickness, confusion, and involuntary movements of the limbs.
Trade names include Eldepryl

Septra *see **Septrin**, below*

Septrin Well known trade name for a combination of sulphamethoxazole and trimethoprim *(see **sulphamethoxazole, and trimethoprim**)*

Serc Trade name for betahistine

Serophene Trade name for clomiphene

Seroxat Trade name for paroxetine

Sertraline
Anti-depressant *(see **anti-depressants** under **Classes of Drugs**)*. Works by increasing the available amount of al brain chemical, 5H-T.

Possible side-effects include sickness, diarrhoea, dry mouth, problems with ejaculation in men, headache, confusion. Best taken with food.
Trade names include Lustral

Sim vastatin
Drug for reducing cholesterol, where diet alone

has failed. Works by blocking an enzyme responsible for manufacturing cholesterol in the body. Taken at night.

Possible side-effects include headache, wind, constipation, stomach ache, tiredness.
Trade names include Zocor

Slo-Phyllin Trade name for theophylline

Slow-K Trade name for a slow-release type of potassium chloride

Sodium bicarbonate
Antacid. A traditional remedy for indigestion, known to generations – often as bicarbonate of soda or 'bicarb'. Works because it is a mild alkali, and therefore neutralises stomach acid. unfortunately, in recent years it has become clear that even such a well-liked agent as this can have side-effects. Too much of it can alter the chemical balance of the body. Do not use it repeatedly, especially if you are elderly, or have kidney, liver or heart problems. Otherwise, the only common side-effect is belching.

Sodium cromoglycate
Anti-allergy drug, first introduced as Intal back in the 1960s, but still very useful against asthma, hay fever and other nose allergies, allergic eye problems and, to a lesser extent, food allergies. Works by stabilising certain allergy cells within the body. Cromoglycate is not an immediate treatment for attacks, as so many patients think. It has to be taken long-term and continuously, in order to give you protection against your allergy. Cromoglycate comes in many forms: for asthma, as an inhaler, nebuliser or a powder contained in Spincaps; for hay fever and similar allergies, as

nose drops; for eye allergies, as eye drops; and for food allergies, as tablets.

Possible side-effects include: in asthma, transient coughing or wheezing; in hay fever and like allergies, nasal irritation; in eye allergies, transient stinging; in food allergies, occasional joint pain and rashes.

Among the vast number of trade names world-wide, the best known are Intal, Cromogen, Hay-Crom, Nalcrom, Opticrom, Rynacrom, Vividrin, and Lomusol

Sodium fusidate

Antibiotic *(see **antibiotics** under **Classes of Drugs**)*. Used mainly for penicillin-resistant infections.

Possible side-effects include sickness, rash, jaundice (yellowness).

Trade names include Fucidin

Sodium valproate

Useful agent in most forms of epilepsy. Alters the level of a natural brain chemical called GABA. Known in some countries as valproic acid.

Possible side-effects include weight gain, loss of hair, fluid accumulation, liver and pancreas problems, also stomach upsets and sleepiness. If taken during pregnancy, increases the risk of spina bifida to the unborn child.

Trade names include Epilim, Depakene, Depakote, Myproic Acid

Sominex Trade name for promethazine

Sotalol

Beta-blocking drug (see '**beta-blockers**' under

Classes of Drugs) used in high blood pressure, heartbeat irregularities and angina, and also sometimes for an overactive thyroid gland.

Possible side-effects include cold hands and feet, sleeplessness, wheezing (alert your doctor at once if this occurs), tiredness, and occasionally abnormal heart rhythms.
Trade names include Beta-cardone, Sotacor

Spironolactone
A 'water pill' or diuretic – in other words, one that helps to clear excess water from the tissues by making you pass more urine (*see **diuretics** under **Classes of Drugs**).

Spironolactone is mainly used to help rid the body of unwanted fluid in cases of heart failure. It works by means of a complex action on the kidney.

Possible side-effects include tummy upsets, disturbances in body minerals, confusion, rashes, incoordination, deepening of voice in women, breast enlargement in men, erection problems.
Trade names include Aldactone, Spiroctan, Alatone

Stemetil Trade name for prochlorperazine

Stilboestrol (diethylstilboestrol)
Synthetic version of female hormone, used for various purposes, including palliation of symptoms in prostate cancer and breast cancer; also used as hormone replacement therapy (HRT) in some parts of the world, particularly as a vaginal cream.

Stilboestrol has an unfortunate reputation, owing

to the disasters which occurred when it was used to try to prevent miscarriage many years ago; many of the female children born after this treatment later developed vaginal cancer.

As employed today, oral stilboestrol's possible side-effects include sickness, water retention, clotting (thrombosis), bone pain, and, in males, impotence and breast swelling.
Trade names include Tampovagan (vaginal pessary combination only), and DES

Streptokinase
'Clot-busting' drug, used in the treatment of serious vein thrombosis (clotting), pulmonary embolism (clot on the lung), and heart attack. Works by altering the complex process through which clotting occurs in blood. Streptokinase has only been in widespread use for a few years, and much remains to be learned about it.

Possible side-effects include nausea, vomiting and bleeding.
Trade names include Streptase, Kabikinase

Stugeron Trade name for cinnarizine

Sudafed Trade name for pseudoephedrine

Sulindac
Non-steroidal anti-inflammatory drug *(see **NSAIDs** in **Classes of Drugs**)*, used against pain and inflammation in various rheumatic disorders, including gout. Best taken with food.

Possible side-effects include fever caused by hypersensitivity – so if you develop a raised temperature, stop the drug and contact your doctor – stomach upsets, sore tongue, rashes,

dizziness, ringing in the ears.
Trade names include Clinoril

Sulphamethoxazole

One of the famous anti-bacterial 'sulpha' drugs.
This group was developed in Germany in the
1930s, and for many years they were of great
importance in fighting infections. In the 1990s,
their importance has diminished, but
sulphamethoxazole is still widely used in
combination with the antibiotic trimethoprim,
under the names Bactrim, Septrin and Septra.
The combination is often prescribed for
respiratory, skin and urinary infections. However,
because of the high incidence of
sulphamethoxazole's possible side-effects (such
as rashes, sore mouth and tongue, and blood
and kidney problems), there is now a strong
tendency for doctors to prescribe trimethoprim by
itself *(see **trimethoprim**).*

Sumatriptan

Anti-migraine drug. A relatively new agent, which
appears to work by opposing the action of the
brain chemical 5-HT.

It is important to realise that sumatriptan is not
for taking long-term to keep attacks away; it is
meant to be taken as soon as you feel an attack
coming on. Do not take a second dose in the
same attack.

Possible side-effects include chest pain and
tightness – in which case you should contact your
doctor and take no more of the drug unless
medically advised to do so – feelings of warmth,
tingling or pressure anywhere in the body,
dizziness, weakness, flushing.
Trade names include Imigran

Suprax Trade name for cefixime

Surmontil Trade name for trimipramine

Sustamycin Trade name for tetracycline

Synarel Trade name for nafarelin

Synflex Trade name for naproxin

Tagamet Trade name for cimetidine

Tamofen Trade name for tamoxifen *(see below)*

Tamoxifen
Anti-breast cancer drug; also used in certain cases of female infertility. Works by its effect as an antagonist to the female hormone oestrogen. There is no doubt that it is a valuable drug, but it will probably be some years before the best ways of using it are fully determined.

Possible side-effects include hot flushes, menstrual irregularities, tummy upsets, vaginal itching, nausea, skin rashes, and sometimes hair loss, water retention, and eye disturbances. Trade names include Tamofen, Nolvadex

Tampovagan Trade name for stilboestrol pessaries, with lactic acid *(see **stilboestrol**).*

Tegretol Trade name for carbamazepine

Temazepam
Drug for insomnia, closely related to tranquillisers such as Valium and Librium. Works by

suppressing brain activity. Although temazepam is effective at putting people to sleep, it will make most patients 'hooked' after quite a short time. So these days, medical authorities recommend it only for brief use, say, to get a person over an episode of sleeplessness after bereavement. Regrettably, the drug has been widely misused by people who have obtained it illicitly.

Possible side-effects include addiction, confusion, lack of coordination, forgetfulness and drowsiness, which may last until the day following dosage, so avoid driving and complex tasks.
Trade names include Normison, Razepam, Restoril

Temgesic Trade name for buprenorphine

Tenormin Trade name for atenolol

Terbinafine
Anti-fungus drug, used in skin and nail infections. Works by splitting the cell wall of the fungus. Tablets may have to be taken for up to six months to beat toe-nail infections.

Possible side-effects include tummy upsets, skin rash, odd taste, joint and muscle pains, headache.

Terbutaline
Anti-asthma drug, also used in chronic bronchitis and emphysema. Works by opening up the air passages. Terbutaline comes in many forms such as aerosol, turbohaler, syrup, spacer inhaler, tablets. Obviously, your physician must decide which form is best for you. Do not exceed the prescribed dose or frequency.

Possible side-effects include tension, headache, trembling, rapid pulse, low blood potassium.
Trade names include Bricanyl, Brethaire Aerosol, Brethine

Terfenadine
Anti-histamine *(see **anti-histamines** under **Classes of Drugs**).* Used to relieve symptoms in such allergies as hay fever, dust mite sensitivity and urticaria (nettle rash, hives).

Terfenadine is one of the 1980s generation of anti-histamines, introduced because they cause little sedation. However, exercise caution if driving or operating machinery and avoid alcohol in case the combination makes you sleepy. Other possible side-effects include hair loss, and – rarely – dangerous irregularities of heartbeat, especially at high dosage and in combination with certain other drugs (notably erythromycin and anti-fungus agents).
Trade names include Triludan, Seldane

Terramycin Trade name for oxytetracycline

Testosterone
This is the male hormone, administered in cases of deficiency, although these are rare. Some doctors prescribe it for impotence, but most medical authorities deny its effectiveness. By an odd quirk of body chemistry, it actually reduces sperm production in the normal male.

Testosterone is sometimes used to try and increase sexual desire in post-menopausal women, particularly in the United States, but this technique is controversial. This hormone and the related methyltestosterone are misused by some athletes to gain muscle strength.

Possible side-effects include oedema (dropsy), infertility, raised blood calcium, priapism (erection that refuses to go down), and in women enlargement of the clitoris, deep voice, hair on the face and spots. Methyltestosterone may cause jaundice.

Tetrabid Trade name for tetracycline *(below)*

Tetracycline
Antibiotic, useful against a wide range of germs. Obviously, one of the tetracycline group of antibiotics *(see **tetracyclines** under '**antibiotics**' in **Classes of Drugs**)*.

Tetracycline is prescribed for chronic bronchitis, some tropical infections, and some pelvic infections in women. For the treatment of acne, it is used long-term: that is, for six months or so.

Possible side-effects include diarrhoea, sickness, and a red rash. In this case, stop taking the pills and contact your doctor. Because it stains developing teeth very badly, tetracycline is no longer given to children or expectant mothers. Trade names include Achromycin, Sustamycin, Tetrabid, Cyclinex, Cyclopar, Nor-Tet, Panmycin, Retet, Robitet, Tetracap, Tetracyn, Tetralan

Theo-Dur Trade name for theophylline *(see below)*

Theophylline
Anti-asthma drug – also useful in bronchitis and emphysema – which works by widening the air passages. It is a long-established, fast-working remedy, but its duration of action is very variable, and is reduced in smokers and heavy drinkers.

Possible side-effects include sickness, headache, stomach irritation, restlessness, lowered levels of potassium in the blood.
Theophylline is available in a multitude of trade-names worldwide. Among the best-known are Neulin, Slo-Phyllin, Theo-Dur, Uniphyllin Continus, Aerolate, Aquaphyllin, Elixophyllin, Lanophyllin, Theophyl

Thiamine *(see **vitamin B1**).*

Thioridazine
Powerful tranquilliser, used in severe emotional disturbances. Works by sedating the brain.
Possible side-effects include fainting on standing up, drowsiness, sexual problems (specially ejaculation happening inward, rather than outward), eye damage.
Trade names include Melleril, Mellaril, Mellaril-S,

Tildiem Trade name for diltiazem

Timolol
Beta-blocking drug *(see **beta-blockers** under **Classes of Drugs**)*, much used in high blood pressure and angina, after heart attacks and in migraine; furthermore as eye-drops, in glaucoma.

Possible side-effects when taken by mouth include wheezing, heart failure, drowsiness, and cold extremities.
Trade names include Blocadren, Betim, Timoptol/ Timoptic Eye Drops

Tofranil Trade name for imipramine

Tolbutamide
Anti-diabetes drug, used in the type of diabetes

which doesn't require insulin injections. Works partly by stimulating the pancreas to produce more insulin and partly by more complex actions. Tolbutamide must always be administered in combination with a strict diet.

Possible side-effects include low blood sugar, tummy upsets, headache and rash.
Trade names include Rastinon, Oramide, Orinase

Trimeprazine

Anti-histamine *(see **anti-histamines** under Classes of Drugs)*. Vallergan is one of the older type of anti-histamine, so it will very possibly make you drowsy. Avoid driving or operating machinery. Other possible side-effects include slow reactions, faintness, rashes and occasionally jaundice (yellowness).
Trade names include Vallergan

Trimethoprim

Antibiotic, used against respiratory and urinary infections, and for prostate inflammation. For many years, this drug was very widely used in combination with sulphamethoxazole *(see **sulphamethoxazole)**,* under the trade names of Bactrim, Septrin or Septra. Recently, concerns about the side-effects of sulphamethoxazole have meant that trimethoprim is increasingly being prescribed by itself.

Possible side-effects of trimethoprim include tummy upsets, nausea, rashes, itching, and blood problems, especially in the elderly.
Trade names include Ipral, Trimopan, Monotrim, Trimpex, Proloprim

Trimipramine

Anti-depressant *(see **anti-depressants** under*

Classes of Drugs). Trimipramine has been widely used to treat depression for around 30 years. It is particularly helpful when some sedation is required – for instance, if you're very restless or have great trouble getting off to sleep – so it is often given at night. It lifts mood by increasing the concentration of two natural brain chemicals, noradrenaline and serotonin. It is not addictive.

Possible side-effects include excessive drowsiness, dry mouth, blurry eye, constipation, difficulty in passing water, disorientation.
Trade names include Surmontil

Trimopan Trade name for trimethoprim

Trinitrin *see glyceryl trinitrate*

Tripotassium dicitratobismuthate
Anti-ulcer drug, often known by the much more manageable names of 'bismuth chelate', or even 'bismuth'. Thought to work either (a) by stimulating healing factors in the stomach or (b) by attacking the germ *H. pylori*, which one school of medical thought now believes to be responsible for many ulcers. Since the mid-1990s, bismuth has increasingly been used with antibiotics such as amoxycillin or tetracycline with metronidazole to try to stamp out this germ.

Possible side-effects of bismuth chelate include dark tongue, sickness, black motions.
Possible trade names include De-Nol, De-Noltab

Triprolidine
Anti-histamine *(see **anti-histamines** under Classes of Drugs)*, used against various allergies, such as hay fever, dust mite sensitivity and

urticaria (nettle-rash, hives). One of the older anti-histamines which produces sedation and lack of co-ordination. Therefore avoid driving and operating machinery. Other possible side-effects include skin eruptions.

Note that triprolidine is often combined with other agents in cold/catarrh remedies available to the public, such as Actifed and Sudafed.
Trade names for triprolidine include Pro-Actidil

Tryptizol Trade name for amitriptyline

Tylenol Trade name for acetaminophen

Uniphyllin Continus Trade name for theophyllin

Univer Trade name for verapamil

Vallergan Trade name for trimeprazine

Valproate *see* **sodium valproate**

Valproic acid
Drug virtually identical with sodium valproate in effects (*see* **sodium valproate)**

Velosef Trade name for cephradine

Ventodisks, Ventolin Trade names for preparations of salbutamol

Verapamil
Calcium antagonist, useful in angina, high blood pressure and heartbeat irregularities (*see* **calcium antagonists** *under* **Classes of Drugs**).

Possible side-effects include constipation, sickness, tiredness, dizziness, flushing, headache, heart abnormalities, faintness. Trade names include Cordilox, Securon, Univer, Calan, Isoptin

Vitamin A

Also known as retinol. Very rarely prescribed by doctors in Western countries, except in the form of multi-vitamin drops for infants. The only real indication for prescribing it in children or adults is the extremely uncommon condition of vitamin A deficiency.

Overdose of vitamin A may cause the following side-effects: enlarged liver, dry hair, skin, blood and mineral problems; possible birth defects.

Vitamin B_1

Also known as thiamine or aneurine. Decificency causes beri-beri. Thiamine (also spelt 'thiamin') is rarely prescribed by doctors in the West, except in cases of vitamin B deficiency caused by alcoholism.

Vitamin B_2

Also known as riboflavine. Deficiency, which is rare in the West, causes inflammation and rawness round the mouth and lips.

Vitamin B6

Also known as pyridoxine. Deficiency causes skin, tongue and mouth inflammation. In Western countries, doctors are unlikely to prescribe this vitamin, except for women with pre-menstrual syndrome (PMS) and also occasionally for women on the Pill suffering from depression (the theory being that the Pill may slightly reduce the vitamin stores in the body).

Overdosage of this vitamin causes inflammation of the nerves.

Vitamin C

Also known as ascorbic acid. This vitamin prevents scurvy. It is very little prescribed by doctors, but some physicians do think that it may help ward off colds, or perhaps make them slightly less severe.

Possible side-effects of vitamin C include stone formation in the bladder or kidney.

Vitamin D

Name applied to a group of chemicals, deficiencies of which cause rickets. This is now very rare, but if you are dark-skinned and live in a smoky city and get little sunshine on your skin, that could mean that your body does not produce enough natural vitamin D.

Do not exceed the prescribed dose. Excess vitamin D can cause sickness, diarrhoea, tiredness, loss of appetite and abnormalities of body calcium and phosphate.

Volmax Trade name for salbutamol

Volraman, Voltarol Trade names for diclofenac

Warfarin

Drug used to stop blood clotting – for instance, after a deep vein thrombosis or a clot on the lung. Works by 'antagonising' vitamin K, which is essential for blood clotting. If you go on this drug, you must have regular blood tests to ensure that you are not having too much – it is very easy for even a slight excess of warfarin to cause very serious bleeding.

Other possible side-effects include rash, hair loss, diarrhoea.
Trade names include Marevan, Carfin, Coumadin, Panwarfin

Welldorm Trade name for chloral

Xanax
For many years the most popular tranquilliser in the United States.
Trade name for alprazolam

Xipamide
'Water tablet' or diuretic *(see: **diuretics** under **Classes of Drugs** at the start of the book).*
Works by making your kidneys produce more urine. Used in oedema (dropsy), heart failure, high blood pressure.

Possible side-effects include tummy upset, rashes, upset in body minerals, blood problems, light sensitivity, impotence.

Zaditen Trade name for ketotifen

Zadstat Trade name for metronidazole

Zantac Trade name for ranitidine

Zestril Trade name for lisinopril

Zidovudine ß
Anti-virus drug; works by preventing viruses from reproducing themselves. Used mainly in HIV

infection. Possible side-effects include anaemia, lack of white blood cells, sickness, loss of appetite, rash, fever, stomach ache, pains in muscles, headache.

Trade names include Retrovir. Also known as: AZT, Azidothymidine

Zimovane Trade name for zopiclone

Zita Trade name for cimetidine

Zovirax Trade name for acyclovir

Zopiclone
Sleeping pill. Used only for short-term treatment of insomnia.

Possible side-effects include odd taste in mouth, tummy upsets, irritability, confusion, lack of coordination, depression, behavioural disturbances, including aggression. It is very important not to drive or operate machinery while taking this drug.

Trade names include Zimovane

YOUR PERSONAL MEDICATION RECORD

It's a good idea to keep a careful record of any medication you've received, especially as side-effects are so common.

This record could be invaluable if you suddenly became ill, particularly if your own general practioner's notes were not available for any reason – for instance, if you were away from home or consulting another doctor.

So, I suggest that you fill in the details of your medication in the spaces on the following page. If possible, put in the dose, and also the number of times taken per day.

If you suspect that you have had any side-effects caused by the medication, describe them in the appropiate column. And please make sure that you tell your doctor about them as soon as possible.

DATE STARTED	NAME OF DRUG (Write down official name and brand name if you know both)	DOSE	TIMES PER DAY	ANY SIDE-EFFECTS?	DATE FINISHED